"It is a privilege to treat people with hands-on therapy and to be able to facilitate healing. It requires skills, but also a continuous quest for anatomical knowledge and understanding."

Jean-Pierre Barral, DO, MRO(F), PT
Developer of Visceral Manipulation
Founder, Barral Institute

1

Illustrator: Christian DellaCorte, Ph.D., CST
Contributors: Christian DellaCorte, Ph.D., CST; Gail Wetzler, PT, DPT, EDO, BI-D

Table of Contents

Ligaments of the Esophagus

Phrenoesophageal (PE) ligaments are collagenous and elastic-fiber structures with interspersed muscle cells found at the lower esophageal junction (LES). Originating from the endothoracic and endoabdominal (transversalis) fascia, the upper leaf inserts into the wall of the intra-thoracic esophagus. The lower PE leaf attaches to the adventitia of the intra-abdominal esophagus. The ligaments position, support, and anchor the diaphragmatic hiatus, helping the LES to maintain gastroesophageal competence.

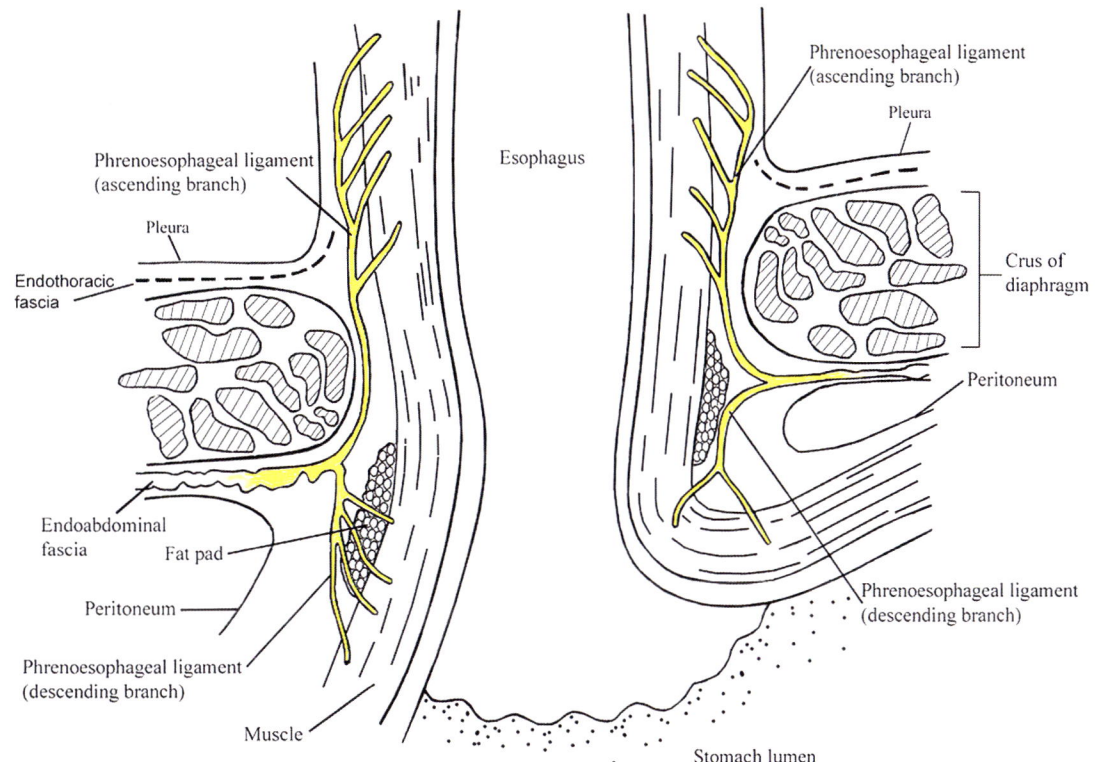

Posterior Peritoneal Wall: Ligament of Treitz

The duodenojejunal (DJ) junction, the terminal intraperitoneal portion of the duodenum, is firmly fixed to the crus of the diaphragm by a band of fibromuscular tissue called the ligament of Treitz—suspensory ligament of the duodenum. When contracted, the DJ junction is thought to aid digestion by widening the angle, allowing movement of the intestinal contents. The ligament is found deep to the pancreas, linking the junction to diaphragm, esophageal hiatus, and L1-L2. The ligament often connects to both the 3rd and 4th parts of the duodenum, as well as the DJ flexure, although the attachment is quite variable.

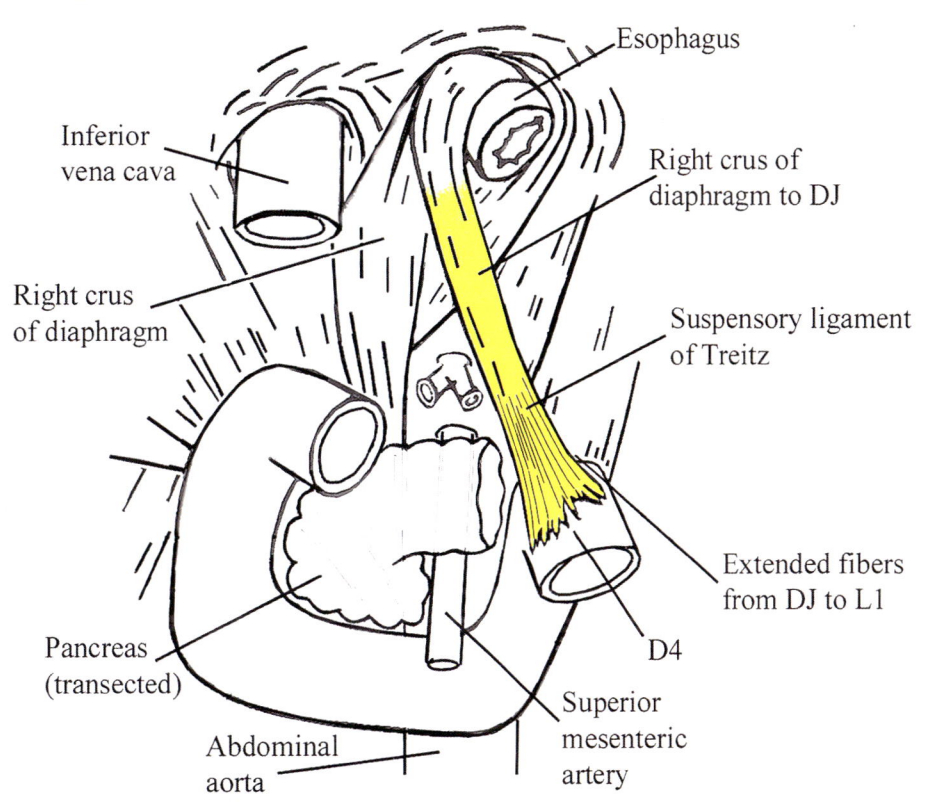

Inferior vena cava

Right crus of diaphragm

Pancreas (transected)

Abdominal aorta

Esophagus

Right crus of diaphragm to DJ

Suspensory ligament of Treitz

Extended fibers from DJ to L1

D4

Superior mesenteric artery

Ligaments of the Pericardium

Anterior support of the fibrous pericardium is accomplished via attachment of the superior and inferior sternopericardial ligaments deep to the posterior surface of the sternum—the upper to the area of the manubrium and the lower to the area of the xiphoid process. The lower pericardium is firmly bound to the central tendon of the diaphragm by the phrenopericardial ligament. Superior support is afforded by attachment of the pericardium to the lower cervical and upper thoracic regions via the vertebropericardial ligaments, a continuous network from the bodies of vertebrae C4-T4. The heart has no lateral osseous attachments, rather it is the function of the lung and pleura that creates a stabilizing pressure for homeostasis. Strain on the ligaments can be transmitted and disseminated, resulting in lower cervical or upper thoracic pain and stiffness.

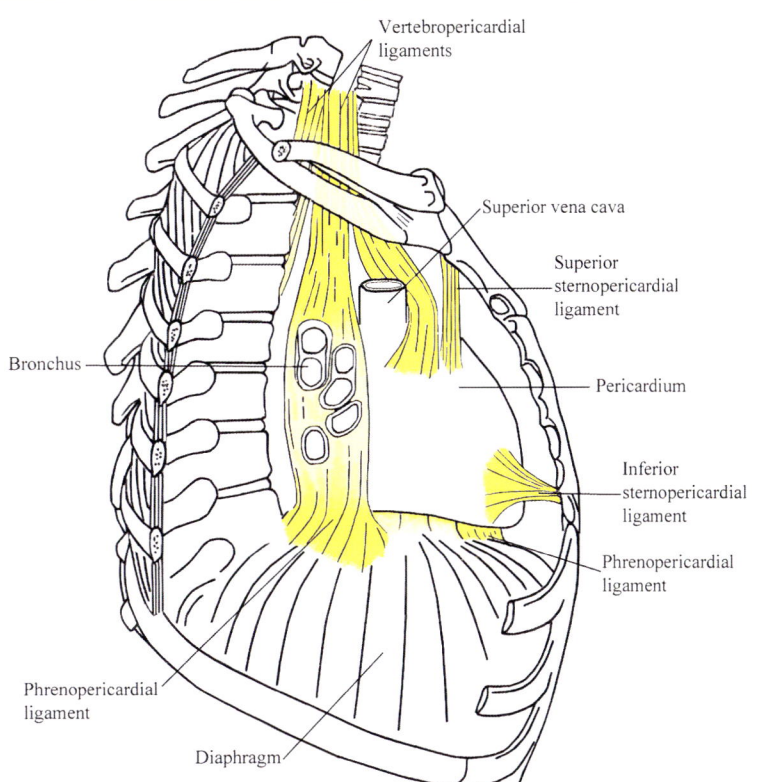

Ligaments of the Pleural Dome

Superior suspension of the pleural dome apex is accomplished via costopleural, vertebropleural, and transverse pleural fibromuscular ligaments to the cervical spine and first rib. In addition to support, these pathways are also able to transmit and disseminate pleural strain to cervical vertebrae. Brachial plexus issues may result from ligamentous tightening due to scar formation as a result of lung infection.

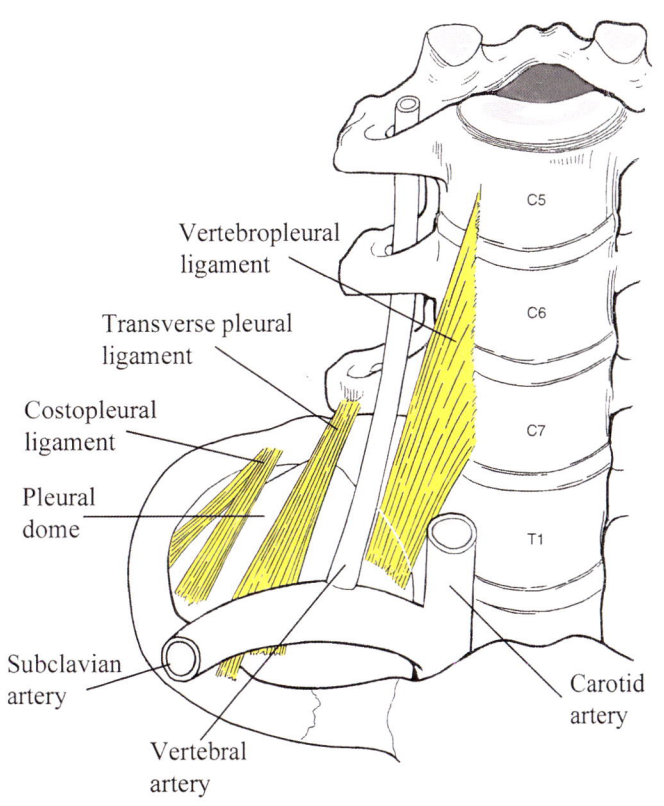

Vertebropleural ligament

Transverse pleural ligament

Costopleural ligament

Pleural dome

Subclavian artery

Vertebral artery

Carotid artery

C5

C6

C7

T1

Right and Left Pulmonary Ligaments

The pulmonary ligaments, ending inferiorly in free margins, are a reflection of the mediastinal parietal pleura extending below the lung root. The mesenteric-like fold loosely attaches the medial surface of the lungs to the mediastinum, approaches the inferior pulmonary vein at the apex, and encompasses intrapulmonary lymph nodes and bronchial veins. The ligaments provide a potential space for lung tissue expansion, for inferior movement of the lung, and assist with expansion of the pulmonary vessels. It has been found in some of the anatomy literature that these ligaments may extend inferior as far as the diaphragm.

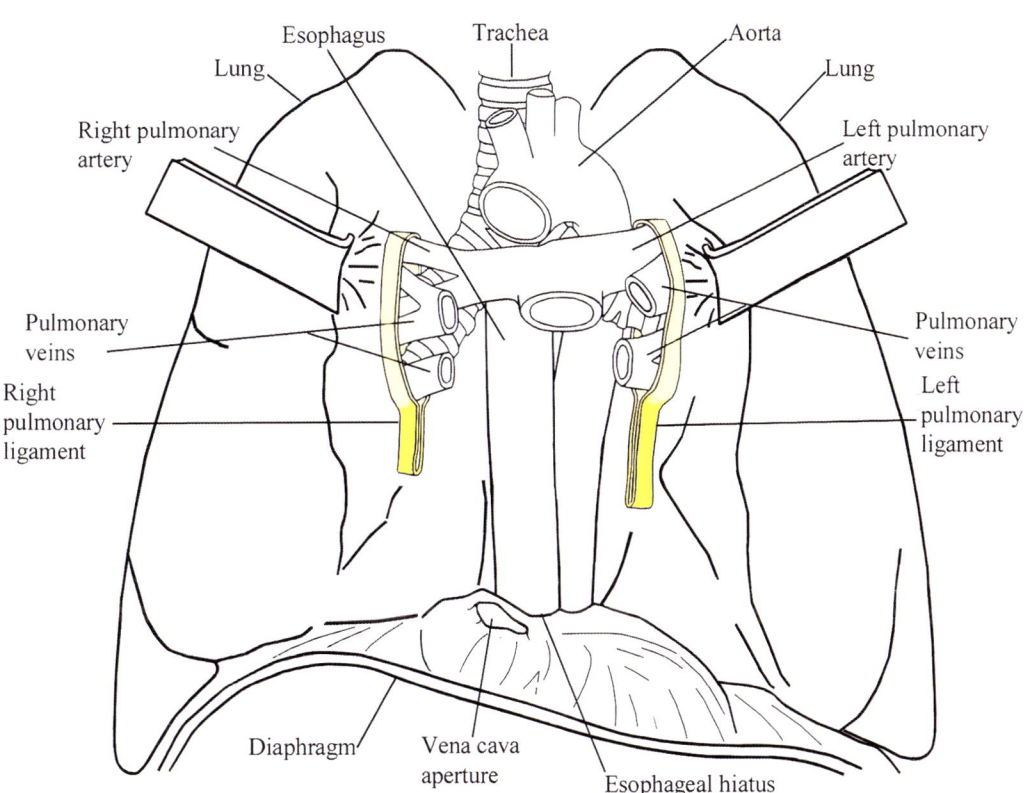

Esophagus

Trachea

Aorta

Lung

Lung

Right pulmonary artery

Left pulmonary artery

Pulmonary veins

Pulmonary veins

Right pulmonary ligament

Left pulmonary ligament

Diaphragm

Vena cava aperture

Esophageal hiatus

Ligaments of the Spleen

The spleen is intimately associated with the tail of the pancreas (pancreaticosplenic ligament), greater curvature of the stomach (gastrosplenic ligament), left kidney (splenorenal ligament not shown), colon (splenocolic ligagment), and diaphragm (splenophrenic ligament) by a series of suspensory ligaments providing direct fixation to the upper left abdominal quadrant.

The phrenicocolic ligament, supporting the spleen from below, is attached to the left colic flexure and diaphragm. Congenital absence or laxity of the ligaments—primarily the gastrosplenic and splenorenal ligaments—leads to excessive spleen mobility, which may result in splenic torsion or a finding of 'wandering spleen.'

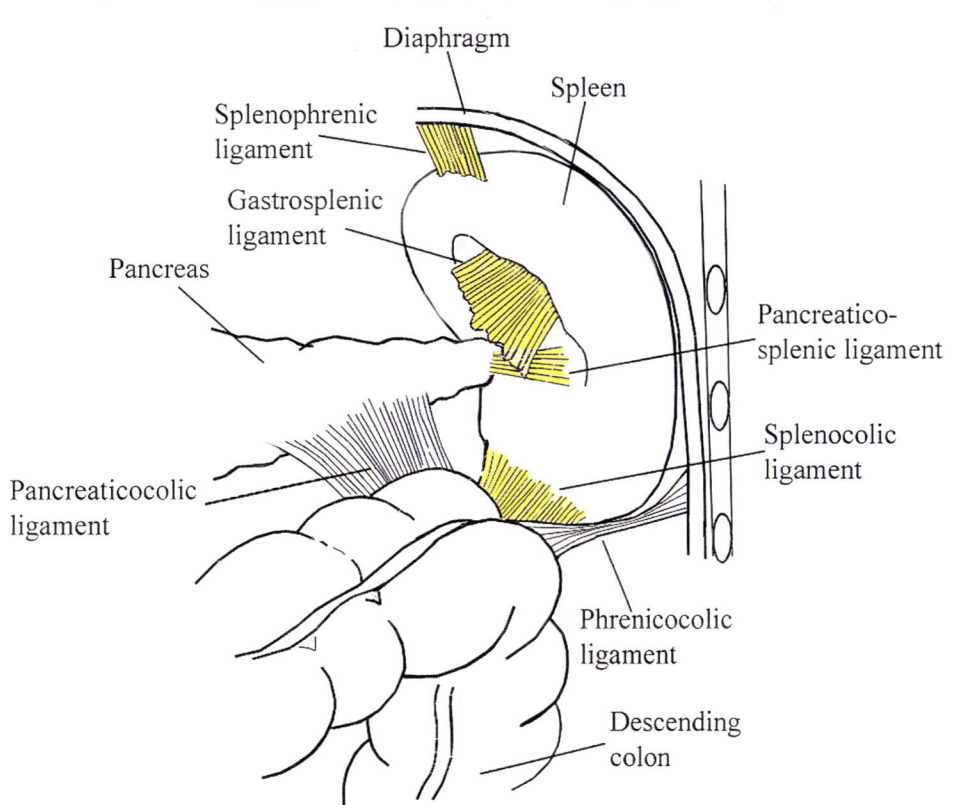

Anterior Ligaments of the Liver

The falciform ligament, tethering the liver to the diaphragm and anterior abdominal wall, is continuous with the anterior layer of the coronary ligament. The two layers of the falciform ligament fan out on the anterior surface, blending with the liver peritoneum as they descend to attach to the posterior aspect of the umbilicus. The fibrous cord of the ligamentum teres—round ligament of the liver—runs in the free edge of the falciform ligament and attaches from the left branch of the portal vein to the umbilicus. In fetal life, the ligamentum teres formed the left umbilical vein whose lumen closes at birth. Although the falciform ligament appears to divide the liver morphologically into a large right and small left hepatic lobe, structural division into a right and left side is due to the portal trinity (portal vein, bile duct, and hepatic artery). See Posterior Ligaments of the Liver page 18.

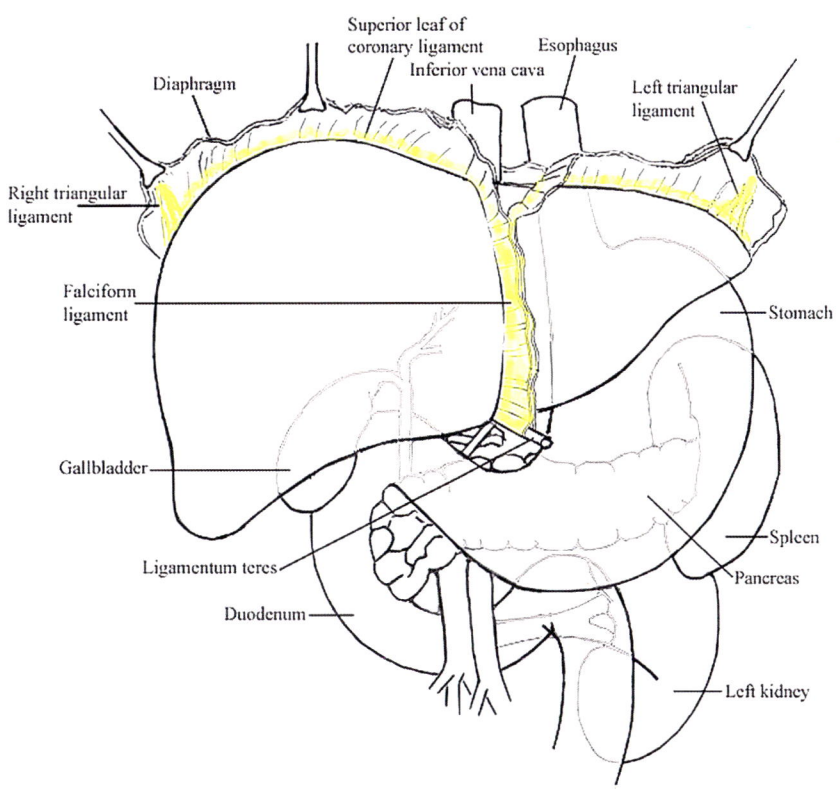

Posterior Ligaments of the Liver

The coronary ligament is composed of superior and inferior leaves, which converge on the right and left sides of the liver to form the right and left triangular ligaments, respectively, suspending the liver to the diaphragm. The two leaves of the ligament are widely separated between the right and left triangular ligaments. At this bare area, the superoposterior surface of the liver lies against the diaphragm without any peritoneal covering. The liver in this section is attached to the diaphragm by fibroareolar tissue, which varies in the density of the fibrous component and is vascular. The dorsal vena cava ligament bridges the posterior right and caudate lobes of the liver behind the inferior vena cava. The ligmentum venosum is the fibrous remnant of the ductus venosus of fetal circulation, which joined the left branch of the portal vein to the left hepatic vein, allowing fetal blood to bypass the liver. See Anterior Ligaments of the Liver page 16.

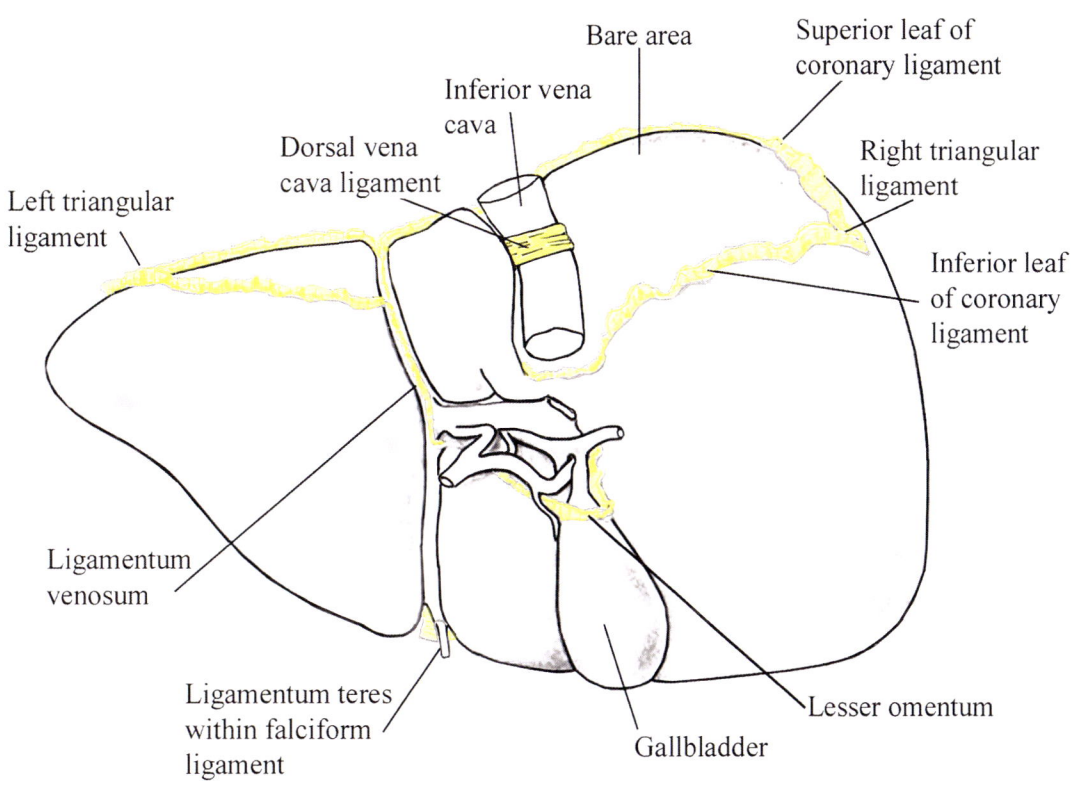

Bare area

Superior leaf of
coronary ligament

Inferior vena
cava

Dorsal vena
cava ligament

Right triangular
ligament

Left triangular
ligament

Inferior leaf
of coronary
ligament

Ligamentum
venosum

Ligamentum teres
within falciform
ligament

Gallbladder

Lesser omentum

Stomach Structural Support: Greater Omentum

The greater omentum consists of the 4-layered omental apron hanging from the transverse colon, and the 2-layered gastrocolic ligament connecting the greater curvature of the stomach and the transverse colon. The omentum usually covers the small intestine as far as the pelvis, and laterally connects from the splenic flexure on the left to the origin of the duodenum on the right.

The omentum is the largest of the peritoneal folds. It is responsible for fat deposition and also is considered a unique immune organ. It isolates compromised areas by wrapping and isolating infected or traumatized regions. The greater omentum also secretes potent immune effector cells/substances.

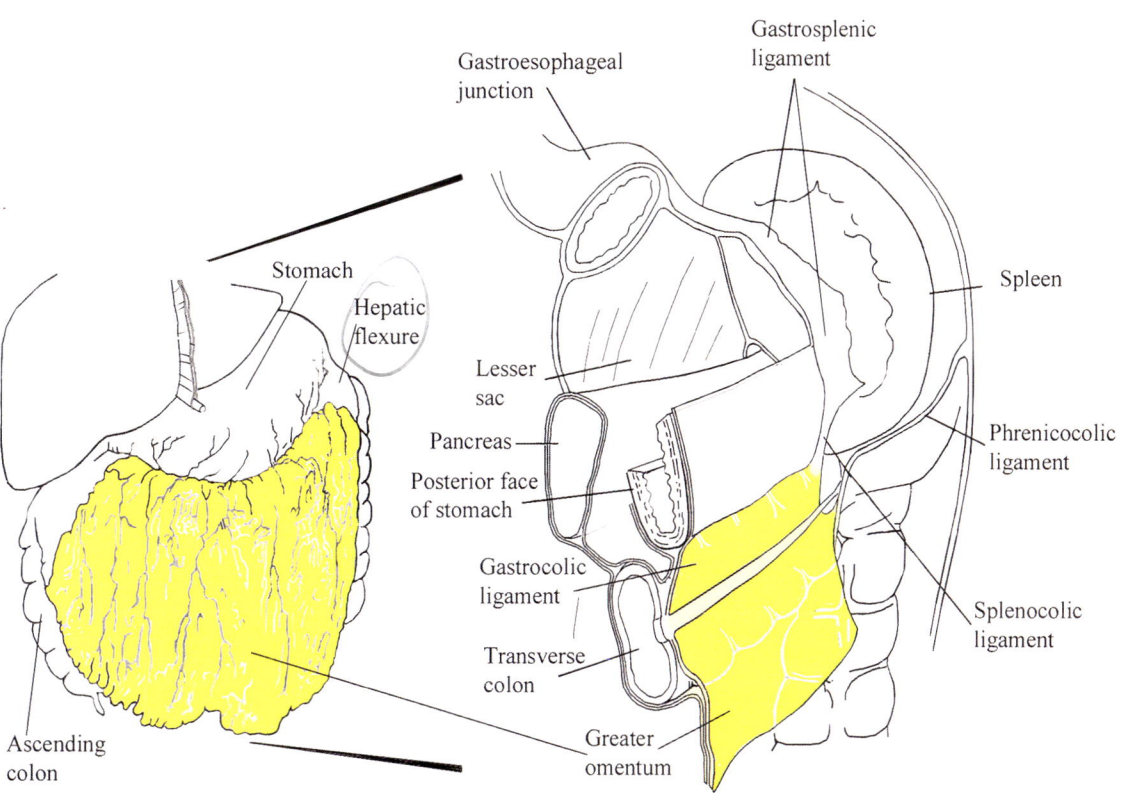

Stomach Structural Support: Lesser Omentum and Gastrosplenic Ligament

The lesser omentum is a thin, double layer of peritoneum extending from the posterior liver to the lesser curvature of the stomach and the first part of the duodenum via the hepatogastric and hepatoduodenal ligaments, respectively. The omentum encloses the hepatic artery, common bile duct, portal vein, lymphatics, and hepatic plexus of nerves. The gastrosplenic ligament extends between the fundus of the stomach and the hilum of the spleen, and is continuous inferiorly with the greater omentum. Literature suggests the gastrophrenic ligament, which is a portion of the lesser omentum passing beyond the esophagus, is considered less supportive than the other suspensory ligaments of the stomach.

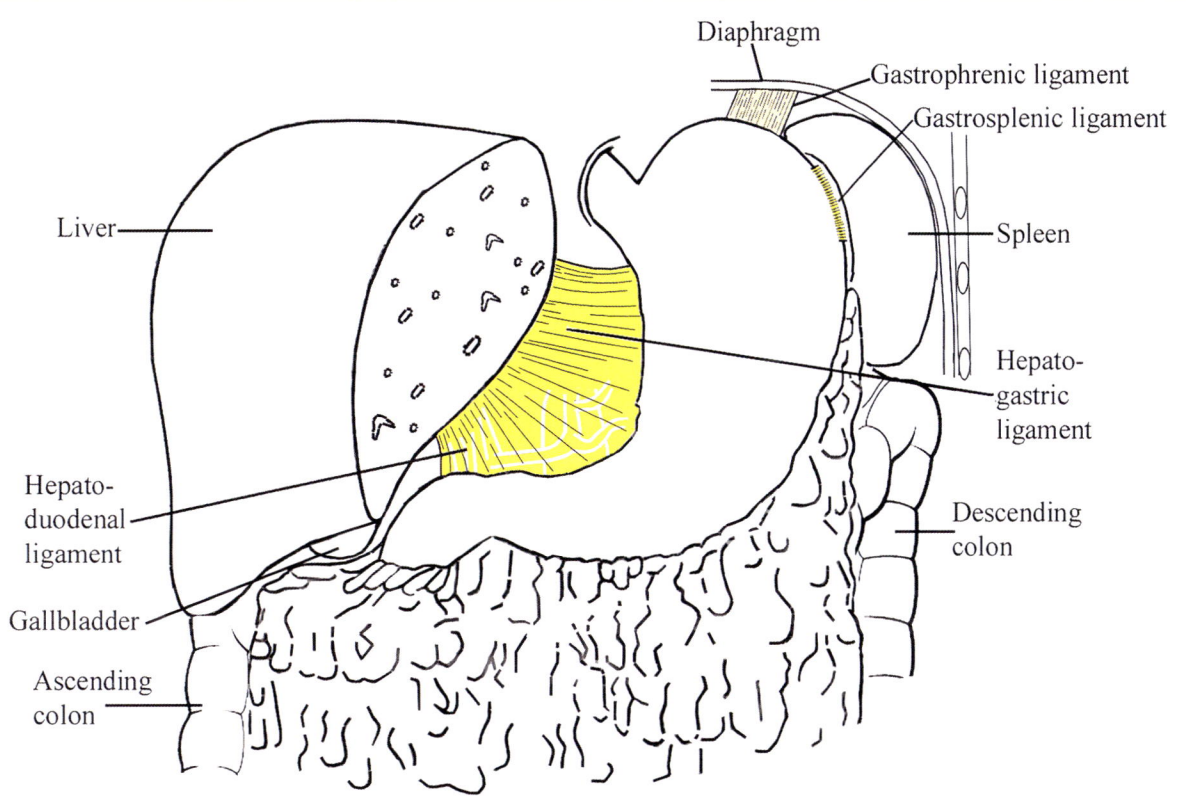

Liver

Diaphragm

Gastrophrenic ligament

Gastrosplenic ligament

Spleen

Hepato-gastric ligament

Descending colon

Hepato-duodenal ligament

Gallbladder

Ascending colon

Transverse Mesocolon: Anterior View

The transverse mesocolon is a broad fold of peritoneum connecting the transverse colon to the posterior wall of the abdomen. The root of the transverse mesocolon extends across the second part of the duodenum and the head of the pancreas to continue along the lower anterior edge of the pancreatic body and tail. Laterally, it is contiguous with the splenorenal and phrenicocolic ligaments. Over the uncinate process of the pancreas, it becomes confluent with the root of the small bowel mesentery. The transverse colon/mesocolon effectively divides the peritoneal cavity, providing a barrier between the supracolic and infracolic compartments. See Transverse Mesocolon: Relationships page 26.

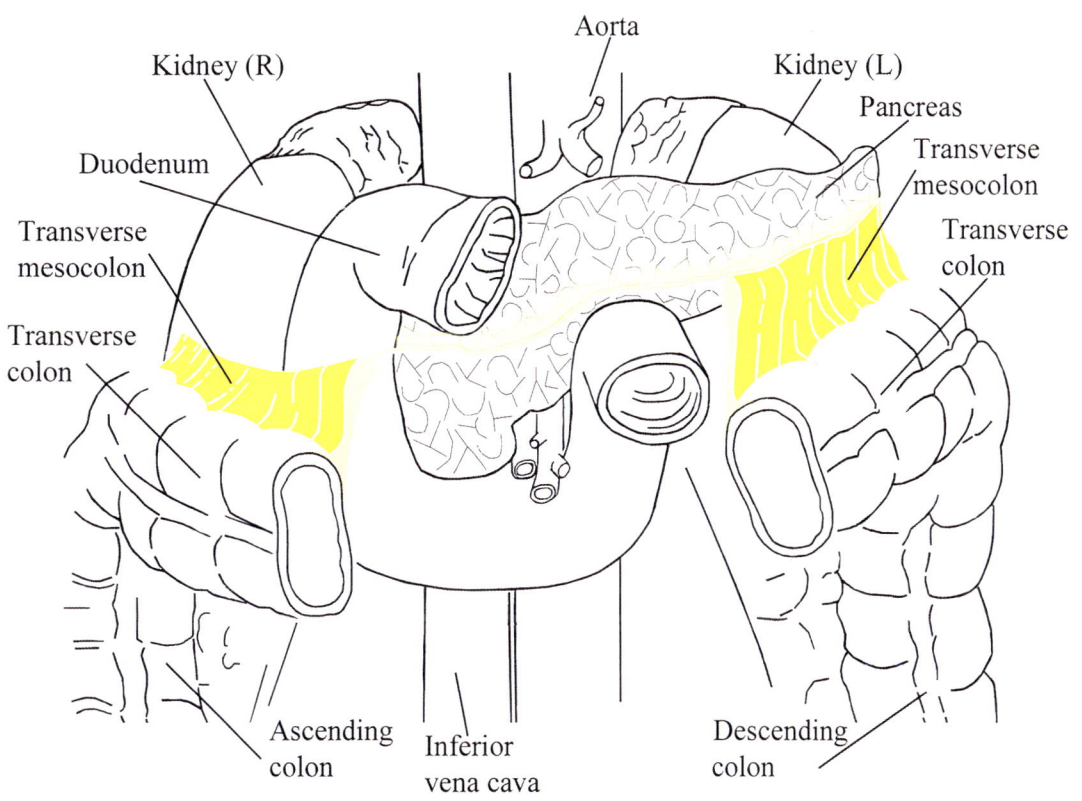

Transverse Mesocolon: Relationships

The transverse mesocolon is continuous with the greater omentum, which separates to surround the transverse colon and joins behind it. The layers continue posteriorly to envelope the anterior border of the pancreas, suspending the transverse colon from the pancreas. The transverse colon is contiguous with the gastrocolic ligament due to its insertion on the transverse colon. See Transverse Mesocolon: Anterior View page 24.

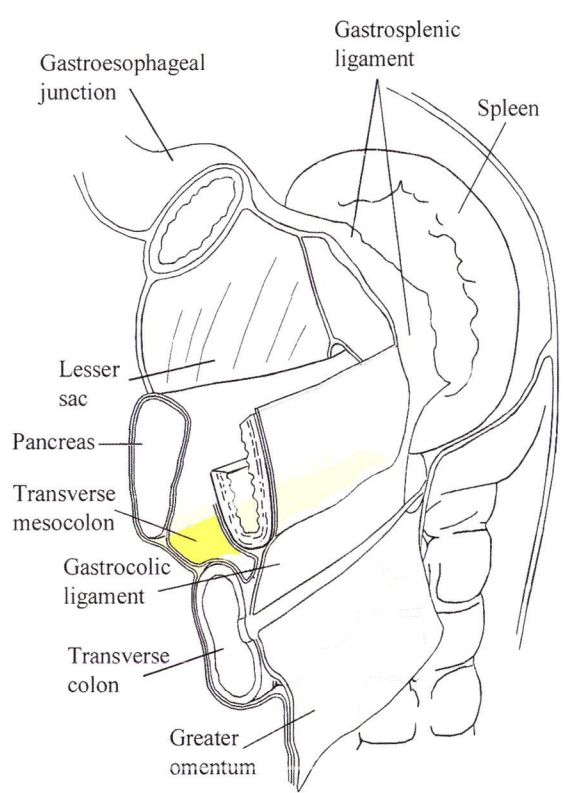

Gastroesophageal junction

Gastrosplenic ligament

Spleen

Lesser sac

Pancreas

Transverse mesocolon

Gastrocolic ligament

Transverse colon

Greater omentum

Gallbladder and Hepatic Flexure

The sharp bend adjacent to the liver between the ascending and transverse portion of the colon is termed the hepatic—right colic—flexure. Superior suspensory colon support is provided by the phrenicocolic, hepatocolic, and cystocolic ligaments. The transverse colon begins at the hepatic flexure and is attached to the undersurface of the diaphragm by the phrenococolic ligament. The cystocolic ligament connects the inferior surface of the gallbladder with the right transverse colon. The hepatocolic ligament originates as an extension from the right side of the lesser omentum and passes from the lower surface of the liver near the gallbladder to terminate at the colic flexure. (Figure adapted from Testut.)

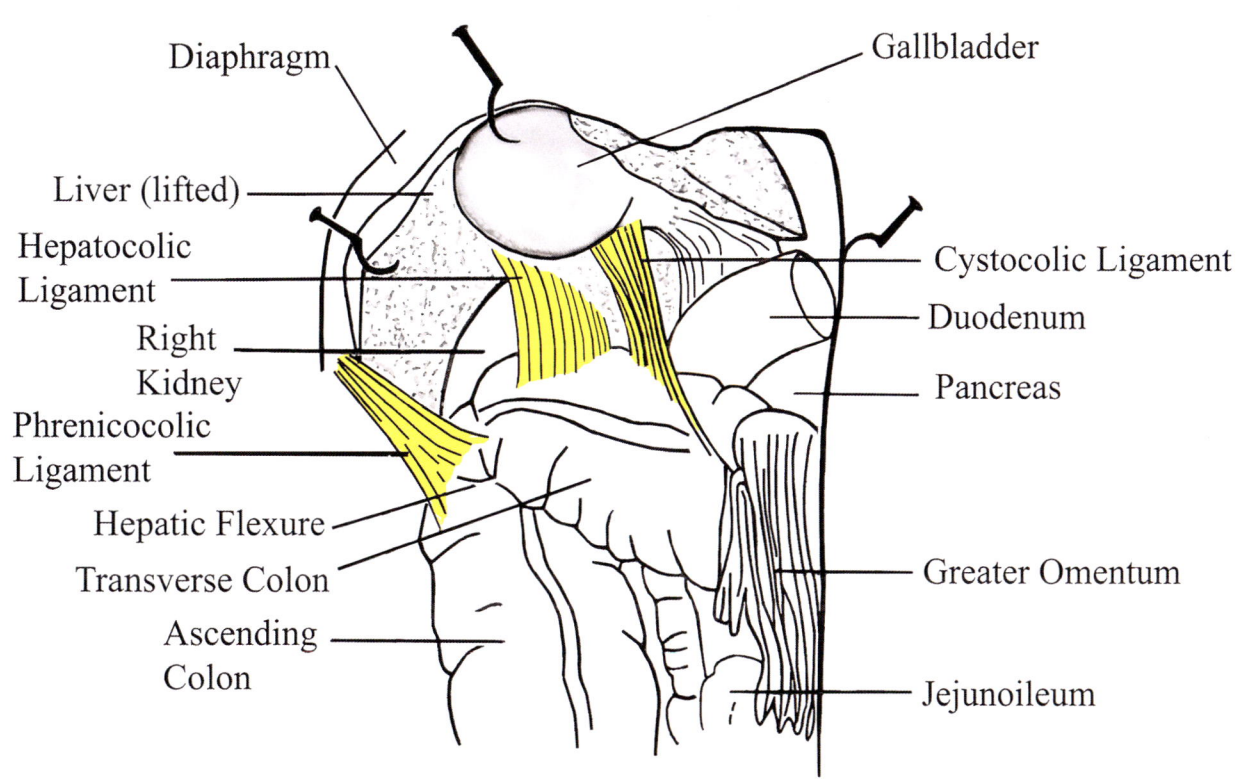

Diaphragm

Gallbladder

Liver (lifted)

Hepatocolic
Ligament

Cystocolic Ligament

Duodenum

Right
Kidney

Pancreas

Phrenicocolic
Ligament

Hepatic Flexure

Transverse Colon

Greater Omentum

Ascending
Colon

Jejunoileum

Supporting Ligaments of the Cecum

Peritoneal folds frequently attach the cecum to the iliac fossa laterally, medially, and inferiorly. These parietocecal ligaments maintain the angulation between terminal ileum and cecum, contributing to ileocecal valve functioning by preventing reflux of chyme back into the terminal ileum, opposing colonic pressures of up to ~80 mm Hg.

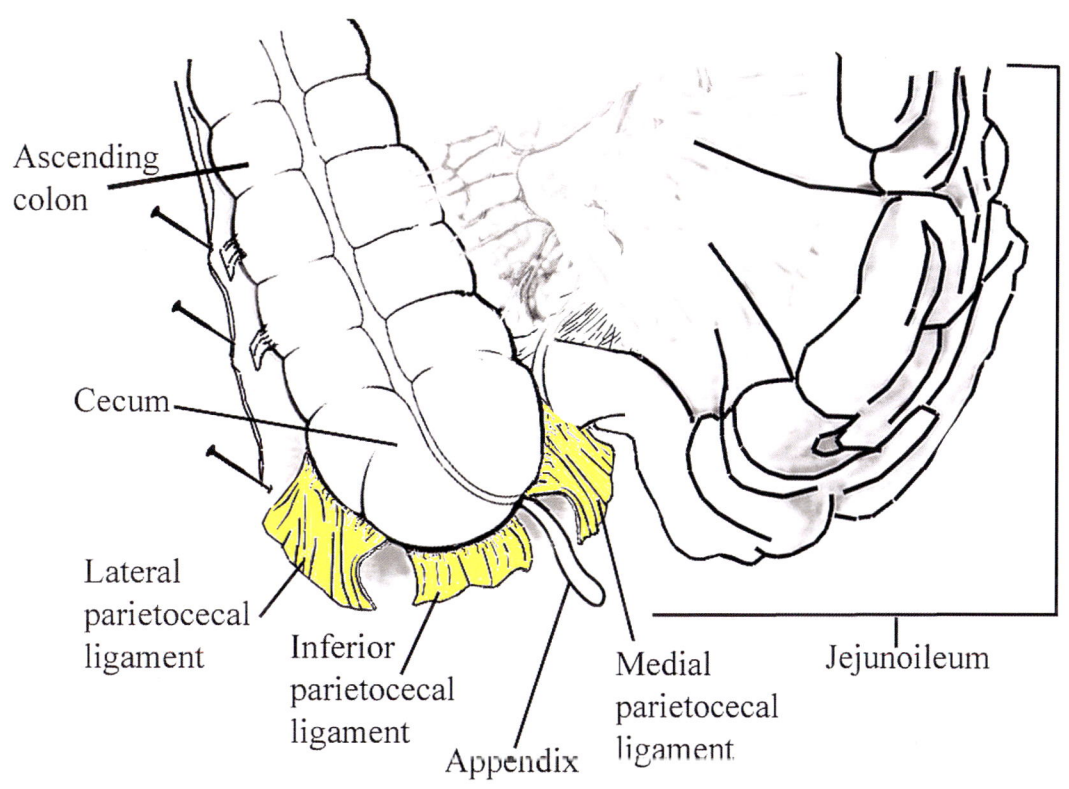

Ascending colon

Cecum

Lateral parietocecal ligament

Inferior parietocecal ligament

Appendix

Medial parietocecal ligament

Jejunoileum

Appendiculo-Ovarian Ligament

The appendiculo-ovarian ligament—ligament of Cleyet—which lies over the femoral branch of the genitofemoral nerve, is a cecum-to-right ovary variant in a higher percentage of women.

Tension produced by the ligament, typically at puberty during the time of rapid pelvic and reproductive organ growth, can present as right medial knee pain.

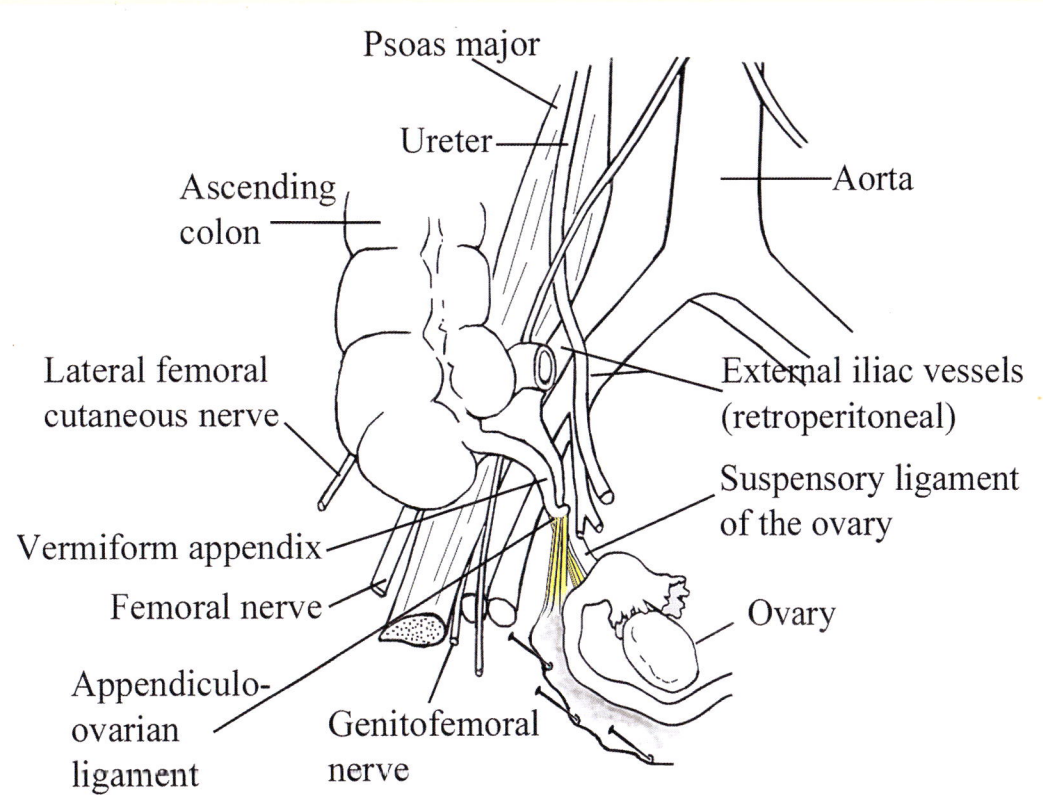

Psoas major

Ureter

Ascending colon

Aorta

Lateral femoral cutaneous nerve

External iliac vessels (retroperitoneal)

Vermiform appendix

Suspensory ligament of the ovary

Femoral nerve

Ovary

Appendiculo-ovarian ligament

Genitofemoral nerve

Fascia of Treitz: Anterior View at L1/L2

The fascia of Treitz—retropancreaticoduodenal fusion fascia—is found at the head of the pancreas, posterior to the duodenum. The presence of the fascia provides both a supportive function and a useful avascular cleavage plane for surgical intervention. See Fascia of Treitz: Transverse Inferior View at L1 page 36.

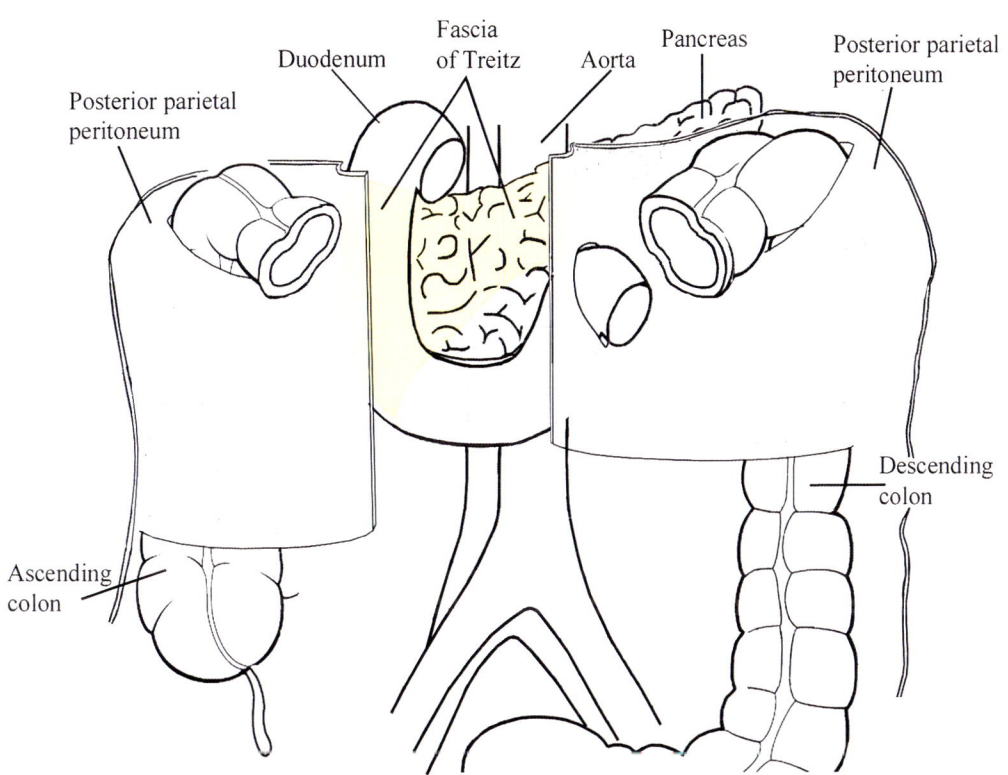

Fascia of Treitz:
Transverse Inferior View at L1

After embryological bowel rotation, the pancreas and portions of the duodenum are surrounded anteriorly by the peritoneum, and posteriorly by the (anterior) renal fascia. The fascia of Treitz is found at the head of the pancreas, posterior to the adjacent duodenal loop, and anterior to the aorta and inferior vena cava. See Fascia of Treitz: Anterior View at L1/L2 page 34.

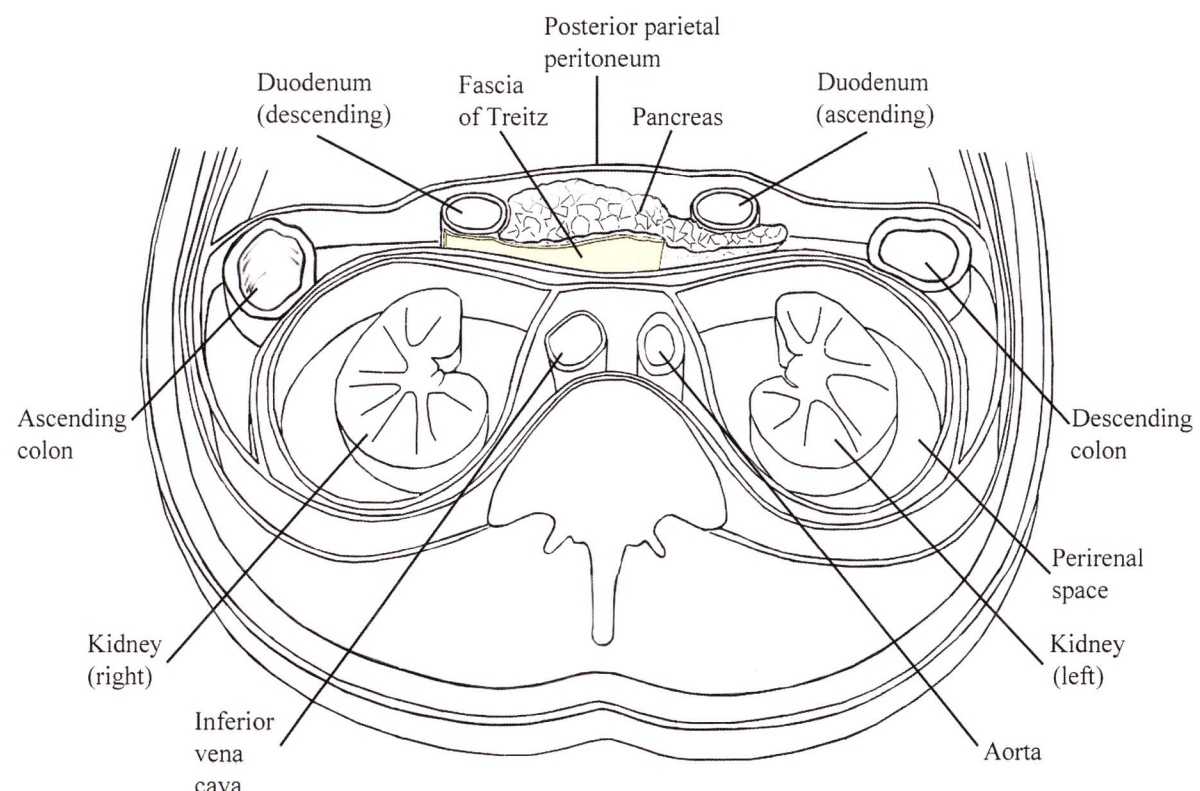

Mesentery Jejunoileum: Superior Leaf

The small bowel mesentery is a broad fan-shaped fold of 'pleated' peritoneum connecting and supporting the 20-25 feet of jejunoileum to the posterior peritoneum. The root of the mesentery measures about 15 centimeters, extending obliquely from the duodenojejunal flexure (left L2 transverse process) to the ileocecal junction, effectively dividing the infracolic compartment into a right and left section. Between its layers it contains mesenteric vessels, nerves, and lymphatics servicing the small intestines. The mesentery presents two surfaces, a superior leaf and an inferior leaf. The superior leaf is continuous with the inner layer of transverse mesocolon and with the peritoneum of the inner layer of the ascending mesocolon. See Mesentery Jejunoileum: Inferior Leaf page 40.

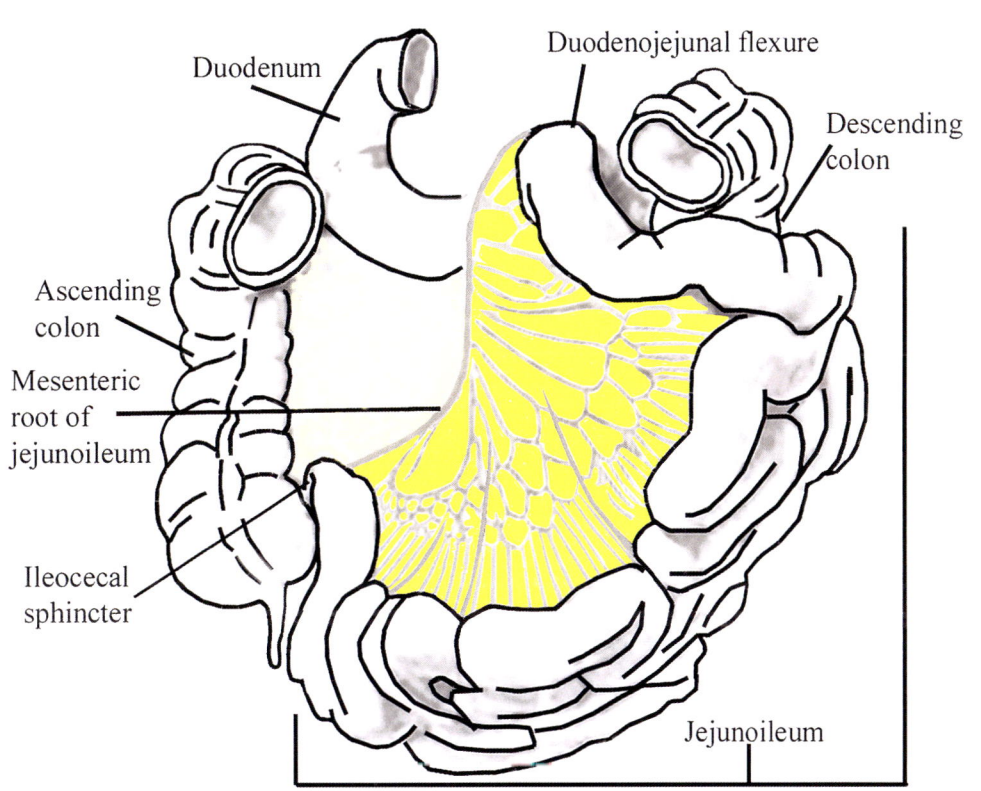

Mesentery Jejunoileum: Inferior Leaf

The inferior leaf of the mesentery is continuous with peritoneum forming the inner layer of the descending mesocolon and the sigmoid mesocolon. It contains mesenteric vessels, nerves, and lymphatics that service the intestines, as well as serving a supportive/stabilizing function. When restricted, the mesenteric root of the small intestine can limit the mobility of the spine as it crosses the 3rd and 4th lumbar vertebrae. See Mesentery Jejunoileum: Superior Leaf page 38.

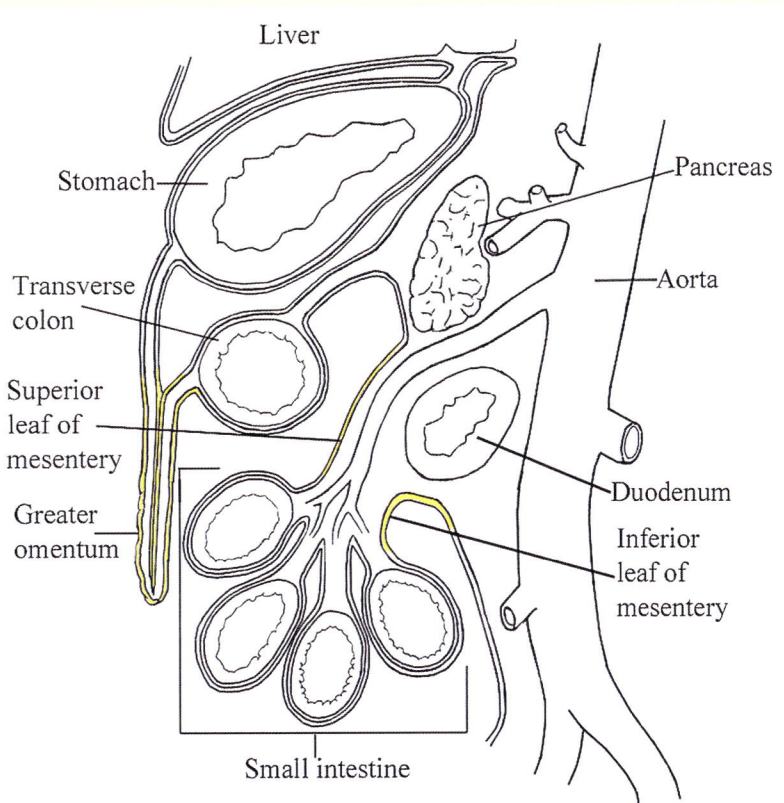

Liver

Stomach

Transverse
colon

Superior
leaf of
mesentery

Greater
omentum

Pancreas

Aorta

Duodenum

Inferior
leaf of
mesentery

Small intestine

Mesentery of Sigmoid Colon

The sigmoid mesocolon, a peritoneal fold, extends from the termination of the descending colon to the commencement of the rectum. Its apex is at the division of the left common iliac artery. The mesocolon connects the sigmoid flexure with the lower portion of abdominal cavity's posterior peritoneal wall and the posterior peritoneal wall of the pelvic cavity.

The sigmoid arteries, superior rectal artery and vein, and the lymphatic vessels and nerves supplying the sigmoid flexure lie between the layers of the mesocolon. The width of the mesocolon permits the greater portion of the sigmoid flexure, when distended, to occupy the pelvic cavity.

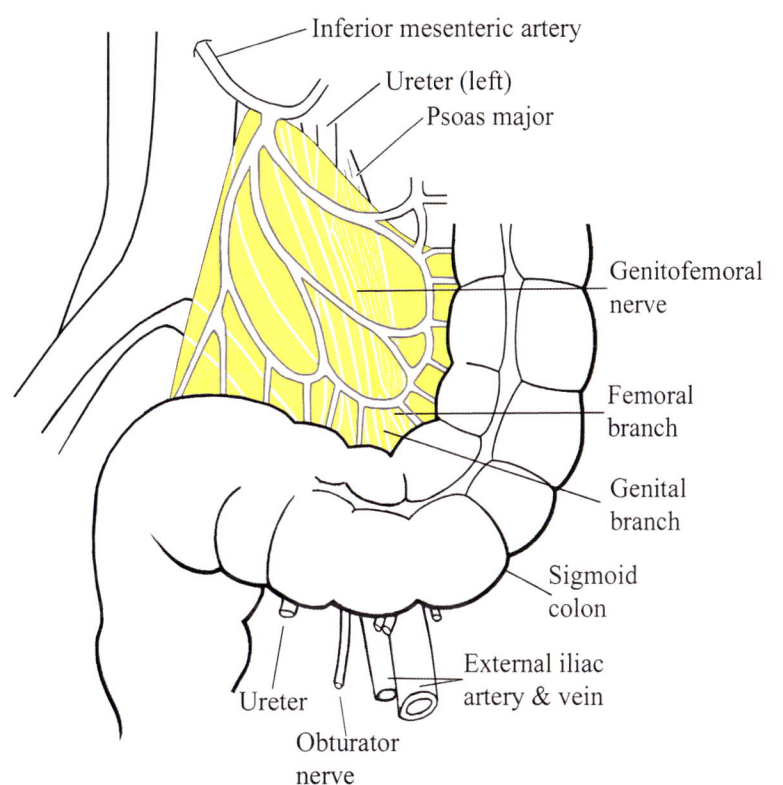

Fascia of Toldt: Anterior View (Peritoneum Removed)

After the ascending and descending portions of the colon come to lie in their lateral positions during embryology, their respective dorsal mesocolons undergo extensive fusion. The anterior and descending mesocolons fuse with the primitive parietal peritoneum and move from an intraperitoneal to a secondarily retroperitoneal position. These fused fascia are named the right and left (retrocolic) fascia of Toldt. See Fascia of Toldt (Transverse Section at L3/L4) page 46.

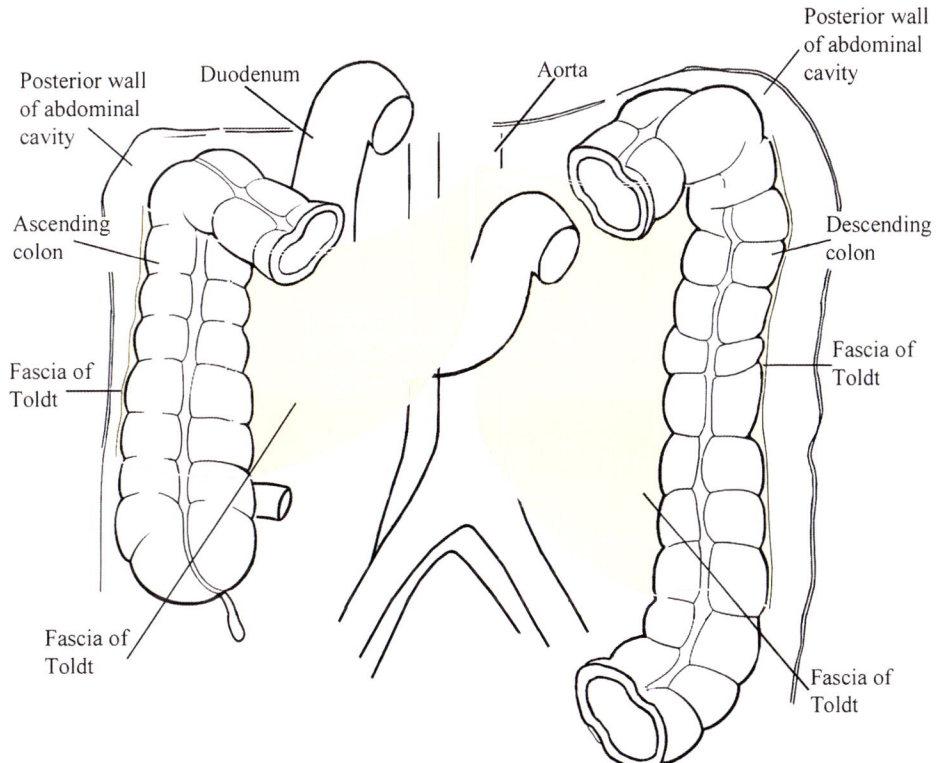

Fascia of Toldt
(Transverse Section at L3/L4)

The right retrocolic fascia of Toldt, situated between cecum and transverse mesocolon, fixes the ascending colon to the posterior abdominal wall near the duodenum and also contains the caudal part of the pancreatic head. The left retrocolic fascia of Toldt lies between the origin of the superior mesenteric artery and the left angle of the transverse mesocolon, superiorly. Inferiorly, it stretches to the upper root of the sigmoid mesocolon. Once the ascending and descending portions of the colon become retroperitoneal, they have peritoneum only on their anterior face. See Fascia of Toldt: Anterior View (Peritoneum Removed) page 44.

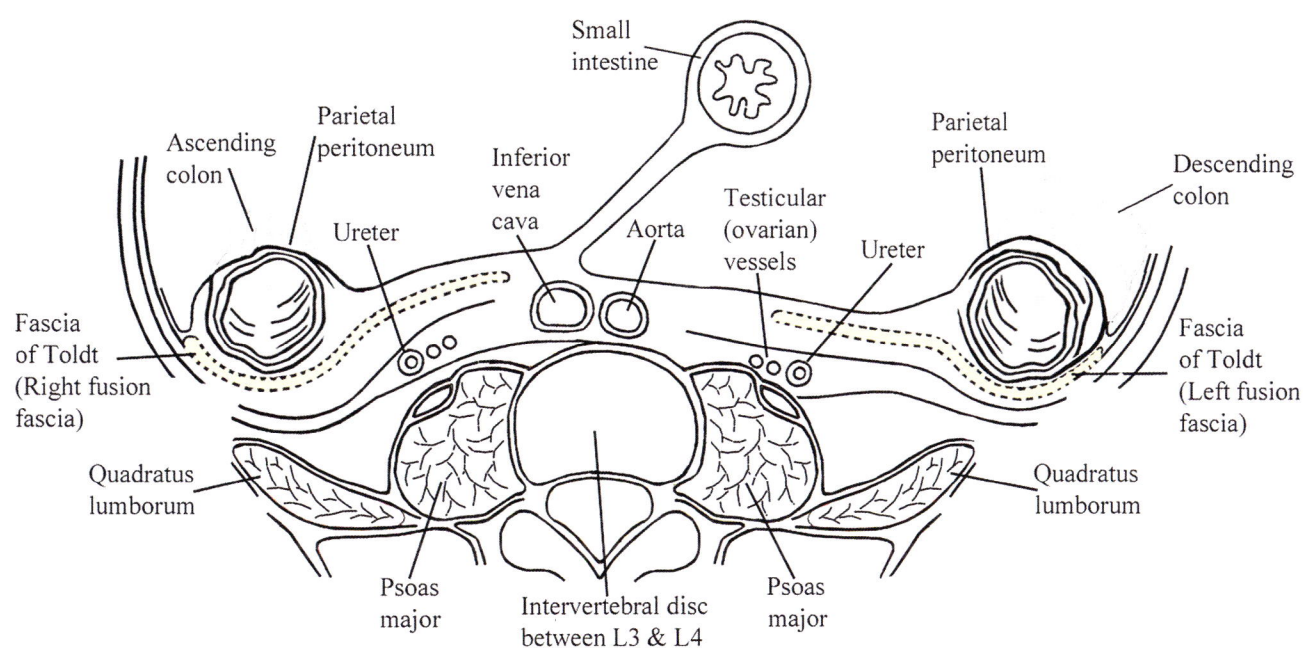

Anal Canal

The anal canal is responsible for controlled evacuation of feces in part due to the action of the external anal sphincter (EAS). Described as consisting of deep, superficial, and subcutaneous sections, the EAS forms a single functional and anatomical entity. The anococcygeal ligament is a fibroelastic-muscular condensation that runs between the presacral fascia/coccyx, and the posterior aspect of the superficial portion of the EAS. Some fibers continue anteriorly, inserting into the transverse perineal muscles at the perineal body—the 'structural beam' of the perineum. The anococcygeal ligament stabilizes the anus and may participate in muscularly reestablishing the anorectal angle during action of the anal sphincters.

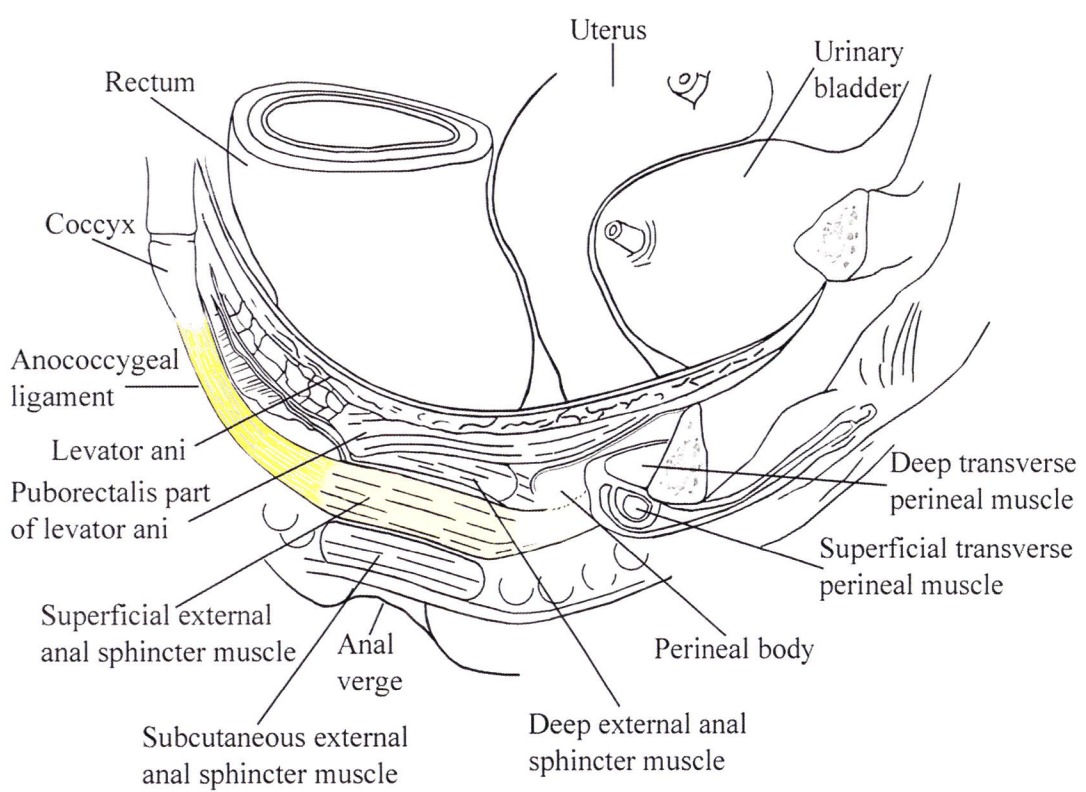

Rectum

Coccyx

Uterus

Urinary bladder

Anococcygeal ligament

Levator ani

Puborectalis part of levator ani

Superficial external anal sphincter muscle

Anal verge

Subcutaneous external anal sphincter muscle

Deep external anal sphincter muscle

Perineal body

Superficial transverse perineal muscle

Deep transverse perineal muscle

Broad and Cardinal Ligaments

The broad ligament is a two-layered peritoneal fold extending from the sides of the uterus medially, to the pelvic sidewalls laterally, and to the pelvic floor inferiorly. Superiorly, the broad ligament encompasses (anterior-to-posterior): the round ligaments, fallopian tubes, and utero-ovarian ligaments. Medially, it encloses the uterus and parametrium. Laterally, the broad ligament envelopes the ovarian vessels, forming the suspensory ligament of ovary, which attaches the ovaries to the lateral pelvic wall. The broad ligament holds the uterus in normal position, maintaining the relationship of the fallopian tubes to the ovaries and uterus. Disorders of the tubes or the ovaries, as well as adaptive shortening from the pelvic fascia due to adhesions or scar tissue following trauma, surgery or inflammation, can strain the broad ligament causing uteral deviations.

The cardinal ligaments—also known as lateral, transverse cervical, or Mackenrodt's ligaments—are situated along the inferior border of the broad ligament, and encompass the uterine arteries and veins. Arising from the side of the cervix and the lateral fornix of the vagina, they provide extensive lateral pelvic wall attachment/support at the level of the ischial spines. Some fibers of the cardinal ligaments interdigitate with fibers from uterosacral ligaments.

Posterior View

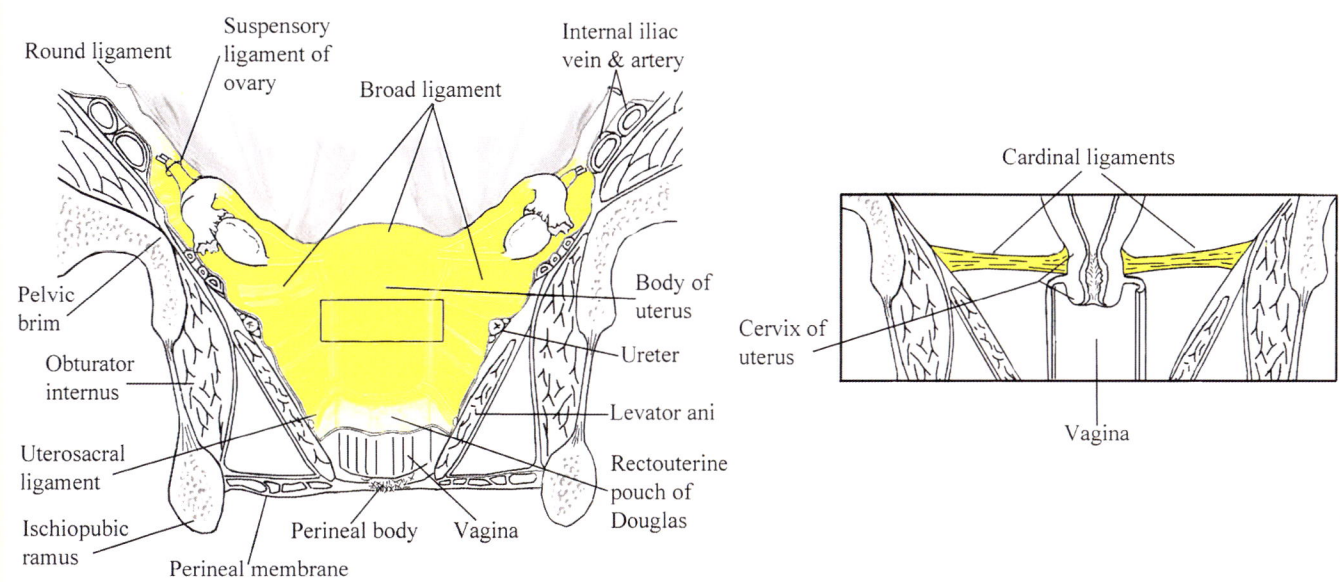

Uterosacral Ligament

The uterosacral ligaments stretch from the posterior aspect of the cervix to the anterior surface of the sacrum, medial to the sacral foramina. The ligaments contain contractile smooth muscle fibers and also encompass hypogastric plexus fibers. They are one of three paired peritoneal ligaments that assist in holding the uterus in place in the pelvic cavity. They are responsible for most of the tension that results in pulling the cervix toward the sacrum resulting in uterine anteflexion or anteversion. Vaginal vault or cervix prolapse can result from lack of uterosacral ligament attachment and support.

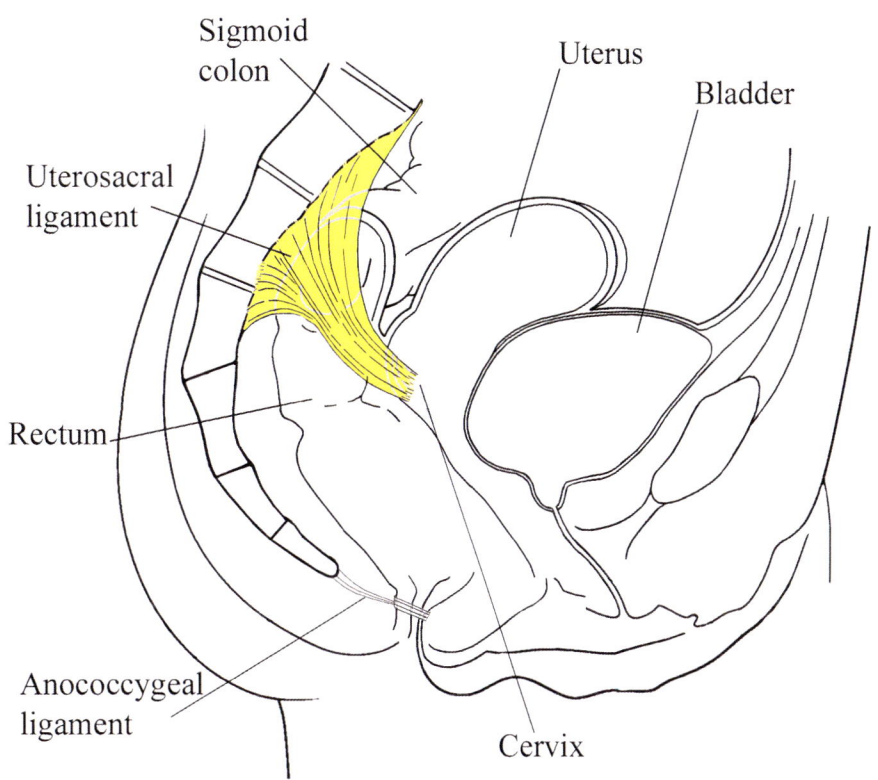

Sigmoid colon

Uterus

Bladder

Uterosacral ligament

Rectum

Anococcygeal ligament

Cervix

Round Ligament

The round ligament is attached to the uterus immediately inferior to the entrance of the uterine tube. It extends laterally and anteriorly to hook around the inferior epigastric artery before traversing the inguinal canal, and terminating in the labium majus. The ligament contains non-striated muscle near the uterus, but is purely fibrous at the labium. The round ligaments function to maintain uterine anterior support during pregnancy.

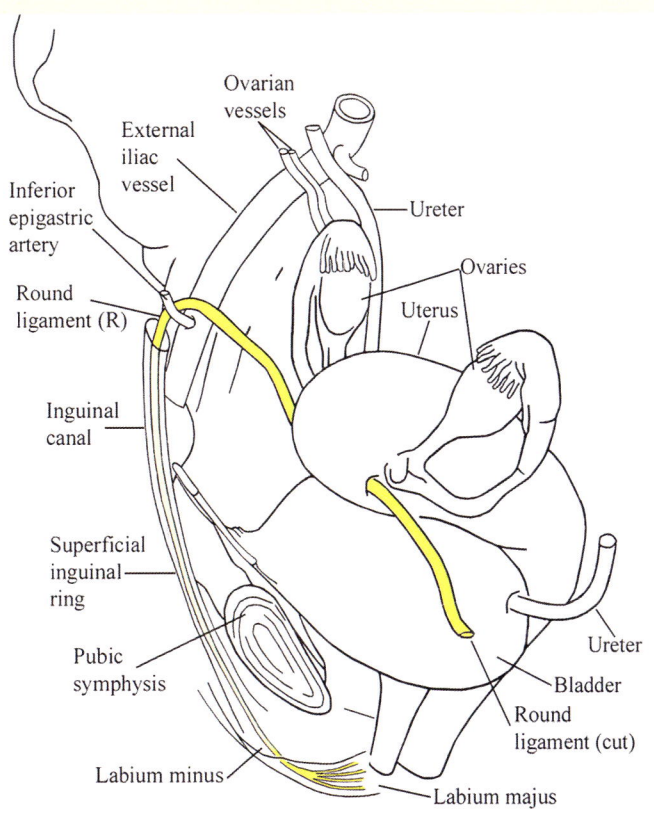

Ovarian vessels

External iliac vessel

Ureter

Inferior epigastric artery

Ovaries

Round ligament (R)

Uterus

Inguinal canal

Superficial inguinal ring

Pubic symphysis

Ureter

Bladder

Labium minus

Round ligament (cut)

Labium majus

Ligaments of the Prostate

Puboprostatic ligaments are pyramidal-shaped thickenings of the endopelvic fascia that insert distally into the periosteum of the pubic symphysis, anchoring the prostate, urethra, and bladder neck. The proximal portion continues with the muscle fibers of the bladder wall into the detrusor 'apron,' a direct continuity of the anterior bladder wall covering the ventral face of the prostate. As it is an important part of the suspensory system, puboprostatic ligament-sparing surgery improves urinary continence after radical prostatectomy.

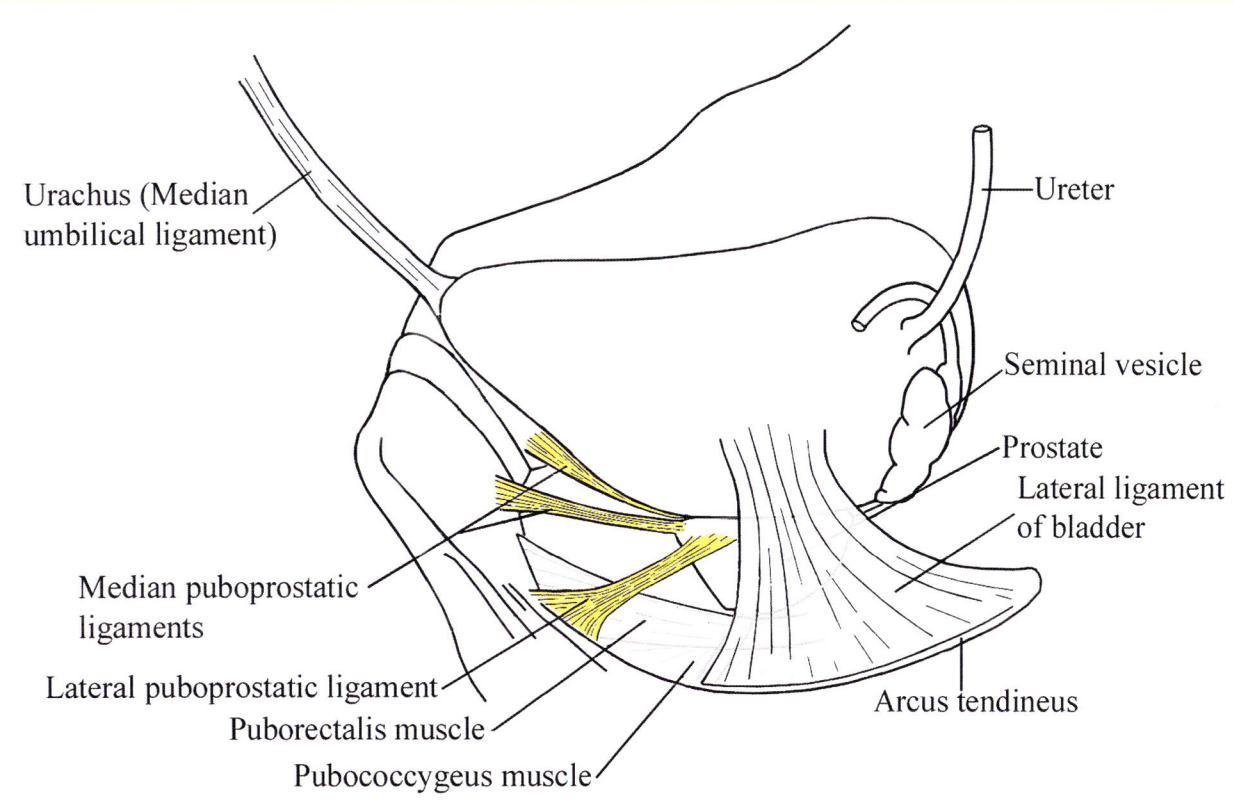

Urachus (Median umbilical ligament)

Ureter

Seminal vesicle

Prostate

Lateral ligament of bladder

Median puboprostatic ligaments

Lateral puboprostatic ligament

Puborectalis muscle

Pubococcygeus muscle

Arcus tendineus

Pubovesical Ligaments

Pubovesical ligaments extend from the bladder neck to the inferior aspect of the pubis bones. Females have two branches: a lateral pubovesical ligament extending from the bladder neck to the tendinous arch of the pelvic fascia, and a medial pubovesical ligament arising from the neck of the bladder and continuing anteriorly to the pubis. In males, the pubovesical ligament is parallel and medial to the puboprostatic ligament, from bladder neck to pubis. Smooth muscle bands within the ligaments are similar in appearance to, and continuous with, the detrusor muscle. Position and mobility of the bladder neck influences continence and initiation of micturition

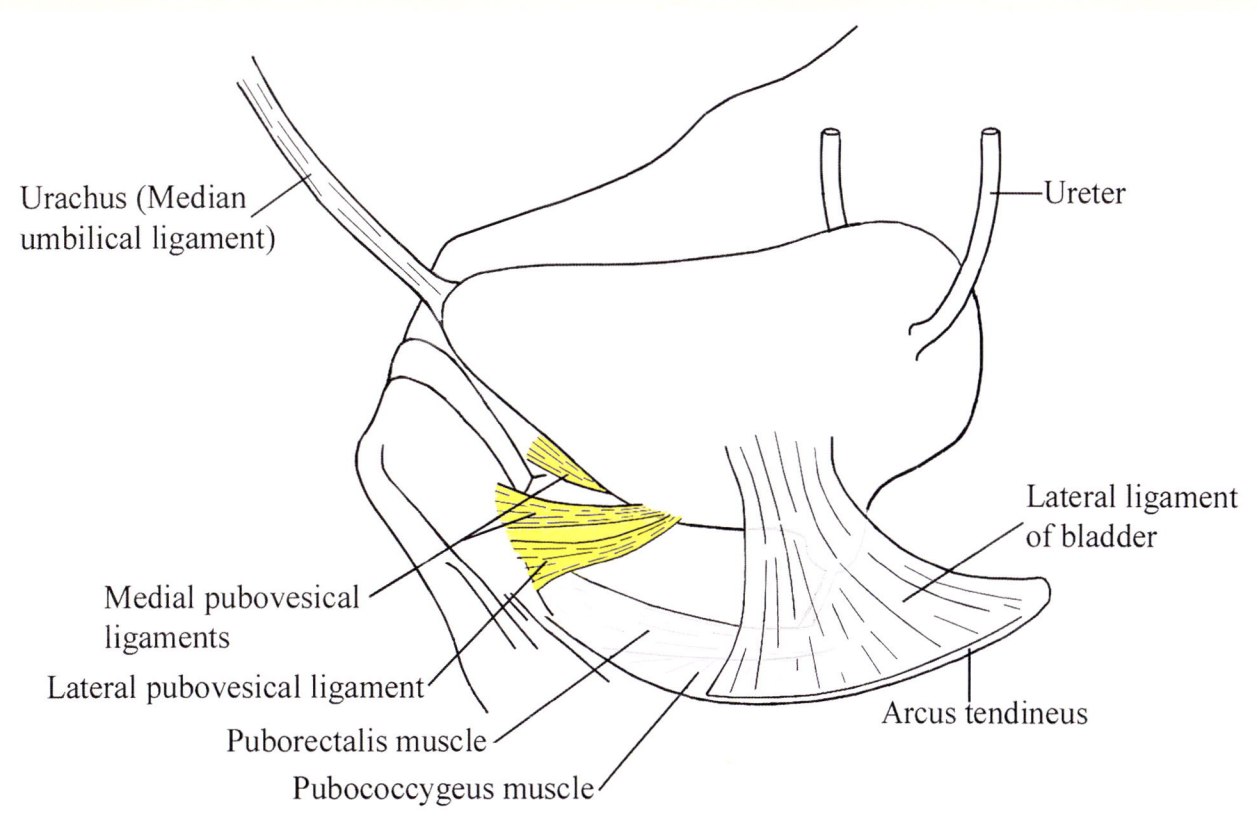

Urachus (Median umbilical ligament)

Ureter

Lateral ligament of bladder

Medial pubovesical ligaments

Lateral pubovesical ligament

Puborectalis muscle

Pubococcygeus muscle

Arcus tendineus

Median and Medial Ligaments of the Bladder

The median umbilical fold runs superiorly from the apex of the bladder to the umbilicus. The fold is formed by the underlying median umbilical ligament, a fibromuscular cord remnant of the fetal urachus. Paired medial umbilical folds pass from pelvis to umbilicus, covering the underlying medial umbilical ligaments, remnants of the fetal umbilical arteries. The urachus and medial umbilical ligaments coalesce to the anterior peritoneal wall during embryologic development forming a superior supportive system for the bladder.

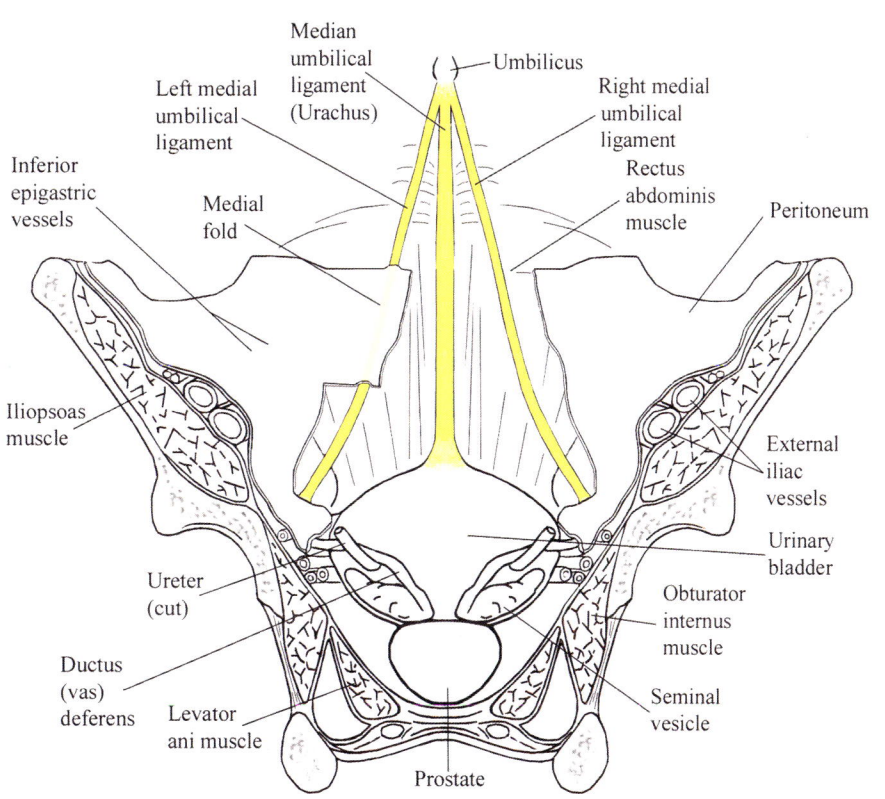